Luís Ângelo Macedo Santiago

Training and de-training on cardiovascular disease risks

Luís Ângelo Macedo Santiago

Training and de-training on cardiovascular disease risks

Influence of training and detraining on risk parameters for cardiovascular disease

ScienciaScripts

Imprint
Any brand names and product names mentioned in this book are subject to trademark, brand or patent protection and are trademarks or registered trademarks of their respective holders. The use of brand names, product names, common names, trade names, product descriptions etc. even without a particular marking in this work is in no way to be construed to mean that such names may be regarded as unrestricted in respect of trademark and brand protection legislation and could thus be used by anyone.

Cover image: www.ingimage.com

This book is a translation from the original published under ISBN 978-613-9-65281-5.

Publisher:
Sciencia Scripts
is a trademark of
Dodo Books Indian Ocean Ltd. and OmniScriptum S.R.L publishing group

120 High Road, East Finchley, London, N2 9ED, United Kingdom
Str. Armeneasca 28/1, office 1, Chisinau MD-2012, Republic of Moldova, Europe
Printed at: see last page
ISBN: 978-620-7-85895-8

Training and detraining on cardiovascular disease risks

Author:

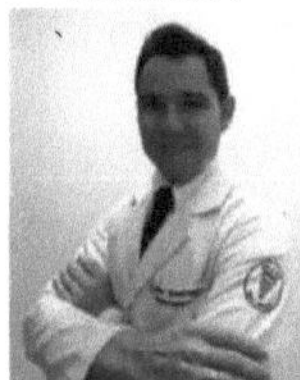

Luís Ângelo Macêdo Santiago

Specialist in Health Sciences and Sports Medicine;

Master in Adult Health;

He is currently a Professor in the Department of Medicine at the Federal University of Maranhão (UFMA).

Author of the book Resistance Training and Inflammatory Responses.

Area of expertise in experimental research in humans and animals, whose line of research is Exercise Physiology with an emphasis on the Adaptations of Physical Exercise in the Neuroimmunoendocrine Axis System.

SUMMARY

Human ageing is a process characterised by both biological and physiological changes with repercussions in terms of altered body composition, with an increase in adipose tissue giving rise to chronic inflammation, indicated by an increase in inflammatory markers. This series of factors leads to cardiovascular risks, increasing morbidity and mortality in this population. Regular physical exercise provides adaptation and beneficial changes to the body, protecting it against various types of disease and causes of mortality, especially cardiovascular disease. On the other hand, its interruption leads to a decline in these adaptations, resulting in the reappearance of diseases and morbidities. This study showed the effects of eight weeks of resistance training, as well as the deleterious consequences of eight weeks of detraining on CVD risk parameters represented by serum concentrations of C-Reactive Protein, lipid profile and body composition in elderly women. The study was experimental with (n = 9) (age 62 ± 2.3). Analyses were collected from peripheral venous blood at Baseline, Post-Resistance Training and Post-Resistance Training. The RT was performed by Combined Series - Bi-Set. The Shapiro-Wilk test was used for statistical analysis ($p > 0.05$). For the group variables, the ANOVA test was performed followed by Tukey's post-test. The correlation between CRP and anthropometric and biochemical variables was carried out using *Pearson*'s correlation ($p < 0.05$). The results show a reduction in fat mass at post-training compared to baseline ($p = 0.02$), while at detraining there was a significant increase compared to post-training ($p = 0.001$). Lean mass at post-training was statistically higher than at baseline ($p = 0.01$). Post-training lean mass was statistically lower than post-training lean mass (p = 0.03). Serum CRP concentrations showed a significant reduction from post-training (1.2 ± 0.3 mg/L) to baseline (2.0 ± 0.3 mg/L) (p=0.008; 40% reduction). Comparing the post-training period (1.2 ± 0.3 mg/L) with eight weeks of detraining (1.5 ± 0.4 mg/L), there was a 20 per cent increase, but no statistically significant difference (p = 0.4). Regarding the correlation between CRP and anthropometric variables and biochemical parameters, there was a moderate correlation between CRP and BMI (r = 0.58), followed by a weak correlation between CRP and the variables Fat Mass, Total Cholesterol (r = 0.49) and Triglycerides (r = 0.37). There was no correlation between CRP and lean mass (r = 0.18). We conclude that the continuity of physical training is essential for acquiring and maintaining good health, otherwise the beneficial adaptations achieved will regress to the initial values, and this depends very much on the type of exercise carried out, as well as the period of interruption in training.

Keywords: Resistance training; Drainage; C-reactive protein; Risk Cardiovascular; Blood test.

SUMMARY

CHAPTER 1

INTRODUCTION

The elderly population is growing all the time, making Brazil the sixth country in the world in the **ranking of** countries with the highest number of elderly inhabitants by 2025 (Netto, 2004). The increase in life expectancy has been studied for many years and by various areas. In the past, it was the privilege of a few to reach old age, but today it is considered a common achievement for everyone (Papaléo, 1996; Caldas, 2003).

Therefore, human ageing is a process characterised by both biological and physiological changes, with repercussions on body composition, giving rise to chronic inflammation, indicated by an increase in inflammatory markers, C-Reactive Protein (CRP), leading to health risks and an increase in morbidity and mortality in this population (Papaléo and Ponte, 2002; Amaral, Pomatti and Forte, 2007).

Among these risks, cardiovascular diseases (CVD) are an important cause of death in developed countries and also in developing countries, where their significant growth warns of their profound impact on both young and old (AHA, 2011, Petersen, Pedersen, 2005). The main risk factors for developing cardiovascular disease are hypertension, high cholesterol, overweight and obesity, diabetes mellitus and a sedentary lifestyle (AHA, 2011).

In relation to the elderly population, who are very vulnerable to CVD, the human ageing process itself, combined with a condition of physical inactivity, has repercussions throughout the body, leaving them susceptible to cardiovascular risks, since a sedentary lifestyle alters body composition with an increase in adipose tissue and consequent alterations in risk markers for CVD (Petersen and Pedersen, 2005). To analyse the risk of CVD, many studies have reported C-Reactive Protein (CRP) as the main acute phase protein and inflammatory marker, and as a risk indicator for CVD (AHA, 2011; Mavros et al. 2014 and Petersen and Pedersen, 2005).

In terms of mechanisms that prevent the risk of CVD, regular physical exercise contributes to mitigating the effects of the ageing process and preventing the development and progression of CVD, reducing co-morbidity and mortality in this population (Petersen, 2005). Recent studies such as that by Santiago et al. (2015), which assessed the effects of eight weeks of resistance training (RT) on body composition, strength and CRP in a group of elderly women, found that RT reduces cardiovascular risk by reducing body fat tissue and reducing the risk marker for CVD represented by CRP. In this way, resistance training (RT) proves to be efficient for metabolic, biochemical and body mass adaptations in individuals who practise it, as demonstrated by Coyle et al, 1984 and Lee et al, 2014.

However, interrupting or reducing this training can trigger a process of deconditioning, affecting performance and reducing the physiological capacity of health determinants. Studies have shown that the abrupt removal of training stimuli results in a lack of synchronicity between the cardiovascular and nervous systems, which can lead to health risks with changes in body composition represented by adipose tissue (Coyle, 1994; Fleck, 2004; Kraemer et al., 2002). Recent studies have demonstrated the effects induced by detraining, such as Nikseresht, Ahmadi and Hedayati (2016) who analysed the deleterious effects of aerobic and resistance training after 4 weeks of detraining and observed that training programmes should not be interrupted.

Although a number of studies have examined the effects of physical training with different protocols on cardiovascular risk parameters in elderly women, this work is important because it determines how long the positive and negative effects of training last after a period of detraining. Therefore, clarifying new information on this issue is necessary, especially for the general population in relation not only to the effects of adherence to training, but also the importance of continuing to practice physical exercise so that the effects achieved do not regress to their initial values. It can be concluded that training has a positive effect on the body, while detraining will lead to a partial or complete loss of physiological adaptations and performance induced by training, particularly changes in markers related to health risks. Thus, the main objective of this book was to provide data on the effects of eight weeks of training, as well as eight weeks of detraining, and their repercussions on serum concentrations of C-Reactive Protein, body composition and biochemical parameters in the elderly population.

CHAPTER 2

THEORETICAL BACKGROUND

2.1 Human ageing

In current times, human ageing and life expectancy have been studied by various professionals and different areas. It used to be the privilege of a few to reach old age, but nowadays it is considered a common achievement for everyone (Caldas, 2003).

Pappaléo (1996) describes ageing as a natural phenomenon marked by important physiological changes, which vary from individual to individual. He also reports that it is a global challenge, responsible for an increase in the demand for care, especially by health professionals. This phenomenon is characterised by both the biological and physiological changes of ageing, where the elderly lose their capacity for biological repair, thus producing ailments that include weakness or deterioration leading to the emergence of various pathologies (Papaléo and Ponte, 2002; Amaral, Pomatti and Forte, 2007).

According to Netto (2004), ageing is defined as a constant and progressive process in which morphological, functional and metabolic changes occur, with alterations in body composition such as an increase in adipose tissue, weakening of muscle tone and bone constitution, loss of functionality, among others, which will lead to a loss of the individual's ability to adapt to the environment, resulting in greater vulnerability and a higher incidence of pathological processes.

Health services will face increasingly intense challenges in the coming years as a result of the ageing population. Zimmer (2001) reports that in-depth studies and the creation of specific public policies aimed at the elderly have been identified as necessary and indispensable for improving the living conditions of this age group. Thus, diseases linked to the ageing process lead to a dramatic increase in healthcare costs, as well as important social repercussions, with a major impact on countries' economies (Nóbrega et al., 1999). Most of the evidence shows that the best way to optimise and promote health in the elderly is to prevent their most frequent medical problems, where these interventions should be directed especially at preventing cardiovascular diseases (CVD), which are considered the main cause of death in this age group. The lifestyle of the elderly, such as sedentary lifestyles, poor eating habits and others, has a direct impact on their health and quality of life, and special attention is needed for this population (Nóbrega et al., 1999).

2.2 Resistance Training

Regular physical exercise offers protection against all causes of mortality, especially cardiovascular disease and type 2 diabetes mellitus in the elderly population, and RT is a widely used method for optimising these events and improving physical performance through muscle strength (Petersen and Pedersen, 2005). In this sense, the increase in muscle strength is an adjustment by the body itself to the overload imposed on it, with neuromuscular changes occurring and allied to the principles of training, the body adapts to this condition (Prestes et al., 2010).

For these adaptations to occur, Petersen and Pedersen (2005); Silva and Macedo (2011) and Lee et al. (2014) report that progressive overloads of effort should be applied during training sessions in order to cause a disturbance in cellular homeostasis and the consequent response to this stress. Overloads can be manipulated through the following variables: load, duration, intervals between repetitions, muscle action, speed of movement execution, frequency of weekly exercises, number of exercises per session, range of motion and combination of exercises in the session, which are characterised in strength training, hypertrophy and muscular endurance (Toigo and Boutellier, 2006; Willis, 2012; Tibana et al. 2012). This overload, according to Barry and Carson (2004); Silva and Macedo (2011); Tibana and Balsamo (2011) is one of the principles of RT necessary for increasing muscle strength, the aim of which is to cause a disturbance in cellular homeostasis and, in response, the body's own adaptation to this stress, causing microtraumas with rupture of the extracellular matrix, basal lamina and sarcolemma.

These microtraumas are of varying degrees in the striated skeletal muscle tissue, resulting in an inflammatory process and constituting a defence process in response to the type of aggression, the aim of which is to prepare the organism to return to its normal functions, re-establishing conditions of tissue integrity and isolating the aggressor organism (Behrendt and Ganz, 2002). This inflammation is considered to be temporary and repairable because it results in a sequence organised by defence cells such as leucocytes and their sub-populations, with the main objective being the cleaning, repair and synthesis of previously damaged muscle tissue (Toigo and Boutellier, 2006).

According to Smith (2004); Lazarim et al. (2009); Silva and Macedo (2011) these repairs caused by overload must respect the rest needed to recover from the acute effects of physical exertion, with positive adaptation of the skeletal striated muscle tissue, in the sense of morphological and metabolic remodelling of the muscle fibres, i.e. the repair process involves the activation of intracellular signalling pathways and subsequent gene activation that can result in changes in muscle mass, contractile properties and metabolic responses.

Smith (2000) highlights this event as a "damage repair mechanism", **where they are** highly synchronised and can basically be divided into three phases: a **degenerative phase** followed by a **regenerative phase,** and a third phase of **remodelling the damaged tissue**. It constitutes a cascade of events in which inflammatory cells promote both damage and regeneration. This is done through the combined action of various factors, such as growth hormones and cytokines, which maintain a balance between pro-inflammatory and anti-inflammatory activities (Tidball, 2005; Gleeson, 2007). It is normally accompanied by a systemic response, called the acute phase response, the aim of which is to adjust homeostasis for tissue repair, i.e. within a few hours of the activation of localised inflammation, the body can show a variety of systemic physiological and behavioural changes, involving various organs and depending mainly on the intensity and duration of the stressor stimulus (De Salles, 2010; Silva and Macedo, 2011).

The first phase of repair is initiated by damage to the sarcolemma with the release of cells responsible for the repair process, in particular prostaglandins derived from eicosanoids that form arachidonic acid and is made up of phospholipids from cell membranes, especially those of the immune system, working to regulate vasodilation (Silva and Macedo, 2011).

Together, these factors enable the influx of inflammatory cells to the injured site, known as diapedesis, and as a consequence, transient leucocytosis occurs. Once active, this will initiate the production of different cytokines, especially IL-6, which stimulates hepatocytes to produce mRNA for the synthesis of acute phase proteins such as CRP synthesised by the liver and fibrinogen (Cermak et al., 2003). The first sub-population of leucocytes to take part in the process will be neutrophils, whose main function is to remove, by phagocytosis, undesirable elements related to tissue damage. This action is considered the starting point in relation to the chronicity of resistance training, as it has subsequent responses in terms of repair, muscle adaptation and tissue synthesis (Tidball, 2005; Gleeson, 2007). Monocytes form the second subpopulation of leucocytes to appear at the damaged site. When these cells leave the circulation and migrate to the tissues, they are called macrophages. Macrophages play a more active role in muscle repair, while monocytes have the main function of removing damaged tissue. Cytokines also play an important role in this process, as they act to recruit and activate fibroblasts that secrete collagen molecules, contributing to tissue regeneration (Zaldivar et al. 2006; Tidball and Wehling-Henricks, 2007).

Silva and Macedo (2011) reinforce this by reporting that all of these TR-related changes in muscle tissue are signalled through the action of cytokines and communicate with other tissues such as the brain, liver, kidneys, endothelium, immune cells and endocrine system, especially the hypothalamus-pituitary-adrenal axis and hypothalamus-pituitary-gonads, to promote the integrated action necessary for healing and repairing the injury.

Another important role of RT is in relation to the metabolism of adipose tissue, especially fatty acids, because during exercise, lipolysis, stimulated by skeletal muscle in these tissues and regulated by hormone-sensitive lipase, activates the beta-oxidation of fatty acids derived mainly from triacylglycerides in adipose tissue and intracellular deposits in muscle tissue. This explains the efficiency and predilection of fatty acids as an energy substrate for active muscle through RT (Silveira et al., 2011).

Recent studies such as that by Santiago et al. (2015), which evaluated the effects of eight weeks of resistance training (RT) on body composition, strength and CRP in a group of elderly women. In the study, RT reduced cardiovascular risks by decreasing body adipose tissue and reducing CRP. In this way, resistance training (RT) proves to be efficient for metabolic, biochemical and body mass adaptations in individuals who practise it, as demonstrated by Coyle et al. 1984 and Lee et al. 2014.

2.3 Physical Training

Just as training develops adaptation and beneficial changes in the body, its interruption leads to a decline in these adaptations. This interruption is known as detraining, i.e. the period in which the exerciser stops the regularity of the exercise programme (Evangelista and Brum, 1999).

Studies have shown that the abrupt removal of training stimuli results in a lack of synchronicity between the cardiovascular and metabolic systems, with repercussions on body composition represented by an increase in body adipose tissue, which can lead to health risks (Coyle, 1994; Fleck, 2004; Kraemer et al., 2002).

It is known that following a physical training programme promotes considerable metabolic changes with a positive impact on body composition, with an increase in lean mass and a reduction in fat weight (Andersen et al., 2005; Melnyk et al., 2009; Mijuka et al., 2004). On the other hand, stopping training results in the loss of these changes (Evangelista and Brum, 1999).

Recent studies have demonstrated the effects induced by detraining, such as

Nikseresht, Ahmadi and Hedayati (2016) who analysed the deleterious effects of aerobic and resistance training after 4 weeks of detraining and observed that training programmes should not be interrupted.

In the same way that physical training causes metabolic changes represented by lipolysis resulting in a reduction in body fat tissue, there are also adaptations in the cardiovascular system, including a decrease in heart rate, an increase in maximum oxygen consumption, an improvement in aerobic capacity and power, resulting in an improvement in cardiorespiratory endurance capacity and, consequently, a reduction in cardiovascular risks (Mujika and Padilla, 2001; Mijuka et al., 2004; Petibois and Déleres, 2003). On the other hand, the deleterious effects of detraining on the cardiovascular system are directly related to an increase in cardiovascular risk due to a loss of metabolic and physiological adaptation, leading to factors related to an increase in heart rate and the accumulation of adipose tissue, with repercussions on risk markers for CVD.

Nonogaki et al. (1995) and Hsueh and Law, (2003) demonstrated the direct relationship between adipose tissue metabolism and inflammatory and CVD risk markers. **Figure 1** shows the metabolic impact produced by a high increase in body fat deposits, which raises the concentrations of inflammatory markers such as C-Reactive Protein (CRP).

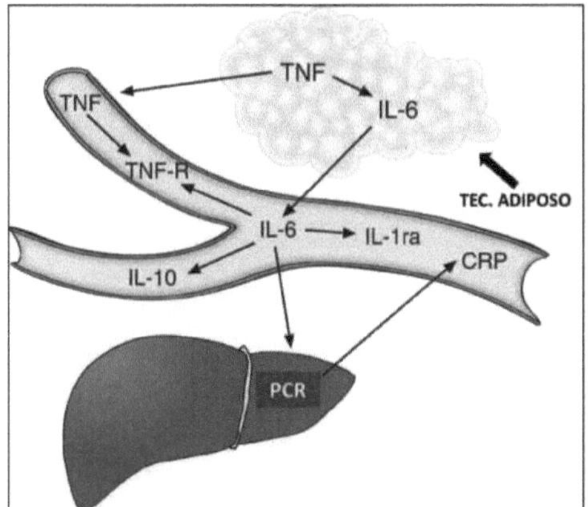

Figure 1: Influence of adipose tissue on inflammatory markers (IL-6, TNF-a and CRP).

2.4 C- Reactive Protein

According to Silva (2009), CRP was discovered at the Rockefeller Institute by Tillet and Francis in 1930, where its factors included the agglutination of pneumococci using reagents that bind to this bacterium's C polysaccharide. Today, it is considered the main acute phase protein and is an inflammatory marker and predictor of cardiovascular disease (Silva, 2009). According to Cermak et al. (2003); Santos et al. (2003); Abbas, Lichtman and Pillai (2012) its production is synthesised by the action of IL-6 from hepatocytes, and it is a direct indicator of IL-6 levels, contributing to the acute phase response and tissue regeneration. Among the various functions attributed to it, perhaps the most important is its ability to bind to cell membrane components, releasing opsonins and eventually phagocytosing and removing these structures from the circulation, promoting tissue regeneration (Abbas, Lichtman and Pillai, 2012).Since its discovery, CRP has been used to assess inflammatory conditions of all kinds and its increase in the body may be related to the response to various stimuli in inflammatory processes, infections and tissue damage and even in adipose tissue. In practice, it is generally used to assess the presence, activity and extent of the inflammatory process (Xia and Samols, 1997; Mosca 2002; Persson et al., 2005; Silva, 2009).

CHAPTER 3

OBJECTIVES

3.1 General

To evaluate the effects of eight weeks of resistance training followed by detraining on biochemical parameters for cardiovascular disease, as well as on body composition in a group of elderly women.

3.2 Specific

A To assess and compare the anthropometric profile of the population studied after eight weeks of training and detraining;

A To analyse muscle strength through load evolution after eight weeks of RT;

Q Quantify and compare the levels of serum concentrations of inflammatory markers CRP, as well as biochemical parameters after eight weeks of Training and Detraining.

CHAPTER 4

METHODOLOGICAL PROCEDURES

4.1 MATERIALS AND METHODS

4.1.1 Characterisation of the study

This was an experimental study. We opted for a pre-test/post-test design with an experimental group, where the participants were randomly assigned (http://www.randomization.com , protocol no. 2538 08/2014, available on 18/08/2014).

4.1.2 Ethical aspects

The study was approved by the Research Ethics Committee of CEUMA University through the Brazil Platform - MINISTRY OF HEALTH - National Health Council - National Research Ethics Committee for experimental research projects involving human beings, under CAEE opinion No.: (10863313.2.1001.5084 opinion No. 372.453/2013).

4.1.3 Inclusion criteria

To agree to participate voluntarily in the study and sign the Informed Consent Form (ICF);

M Women aged at least 60 and no more than 70;

N Not having taken part in any structured and monitored Resistance Training programme in the last 6 months;

P Non-smoking participants who influence the performance imposed by the Training;

P Participants who do not characterise any degree of Obesity, **according to WHO,(1998) in BMI and WHR parameters (BMI=< 30kg/m^2 and WHR= <1.00).**

4.1.4 Exclusion criteria

P Participants with uncontrolled systemic arterial hypertension, i.e. who are not taking medication to control it;

P Participants with uncontrolled diabetes mellitus, i.e. who are not being controlled by insulin: To control these criteria, a Targeted Anamnesis Questionnaire (Appendix 2) was used;

P Participants with changes in the total number of leucocytes that indicate acute infectious processes in the biochemical analysis of the leucogram;

P Participants who attended less than 85% of the sessions over the eight weeks of the training programme.

4.1.5 Sample selection

This is a non-probabilistic sample, and initially a list of names and contacts of elderly women aged between 60 and 70 was requested from the Integrated University of the Third Age - UNITI-UFMA. Based on the telephone contacts provided, the participants were invited to take part in the project. After this stage, participants who had not taken part in any other structured TR programme in the last six months were selected. A meeting was then scheduled for further clarification of the project's logistics, the delivery of the timetable with all the stages carried out, together with the signing of the informed consent form - ICF, so that the days, times and place for the anthropometry assessments and blood collections could be scheduled. The participants were instructed on anthropometric and blood data collection and informed that all the procedures would be carried out in two stages, Pre and Post eight weeks of Training and Detraining.

4.1.6 Experimental design

In this study we opted for a pre-test/post-test design with a control group, where the participants were randomly assigned *(http://www. randomisation. com*, protocol no. 2538 08/2014, available on 18/08/2014). The group was pre-tested (PRE) and posttested (POST) in eight weeks of Training and Detraining. The Training group underwent RT, as well as the interruption phase of this Training, called Detraining. The initial sample consisted of nine participants who underwent anthropometric assessment and blood sampling. After eight weeks, the participants returned to the laboratory and a new anthropometric assessment and blood collection were carried out.

Figure 2

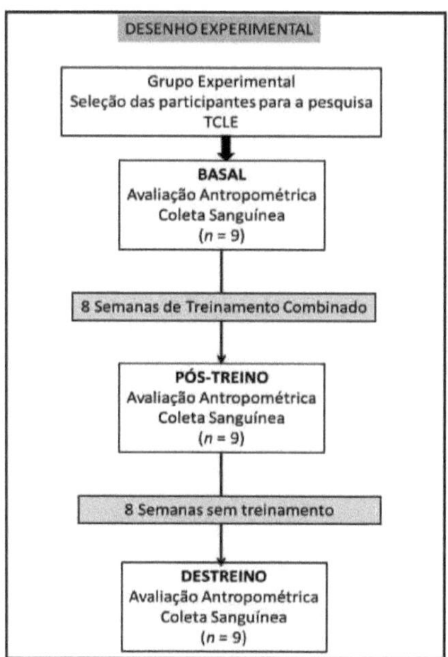

Figure 2 - Flowchart of the activities carried out during the experimental research

CHAPTER 5

Resistance Training Programme

The RT programme was carried out at the Maranhão Physiology and Exercise Prescription Laboratory (LAFIPEMA), located in the Sports Centre of the Physical Education Department at the Federal University of Maranhão (UFMA), starting in August and ending in December 2014.

Initially, the participants underwent a week of familiarisation with RT, consisting of two sets of 15 submaximal repetitions, with the aim of getting to know the exercises and their respective executions and promoting neuromuscular adaptations, thus avoiding the excessive onset of Late Onset Muscle Pain (DOMS). During familiarisation, the participants were instructed to perform the movements at a speed lasting three seconds for each movement, with 1.5 seconds for the

concentric phase and 1.5 seconds for the eccentric phase, controlled by visual and verbal commands to standardise movement angles (ACSM, 2011).

The RT programme was structured after a critical analysis of the recommendations for prescribing resistance training for the elderly (AHA, 2007; ACSM, 2011; Tibana et al., 2012; Hyun-Sub Kim and Dae-Geun Kim, 2013), which was carried out on weight training equipment over eight weeks. The training system adopted was Combined Series - Bi-Set, alternated by segment, as shown in **Table 1**, which consisted of performing two exercises without a time interval for different muscle groups, lower limbs and upper limbs and after performing them, there is an interval for the second pass, after repeating the interval, the third pass begins, where it consisted of 8 exercises, namely: Seated leg press, biceps curl on the low pulley, extension chair, seated bench press, flexor table, open front pulley, seated leg press, triceps pulley.

The intensity of the training was determined by the zone of maximum repetitions (RM) between 8 and 12 RM, prioritising muscle hypertrophy training. To control the training protocol, an individualised programme sheet containing all the exercises in the training programme was used. Two criteria were used to control and increase the intensity (load-kg): 1) The BORG Effort Perception Scale was used to determine the load increase according to the intensity of effort reported by the participants; 2) All the participants carried out their RT programme within a maximum repetition zone of between 8 and 12 repetitions, so every time the participants exceeded the limits of this zone, a new load increase took place to keep them back within the established zone.

The daily sessions were timed and lasted 45-55 min per session. For better control of the programme, all training sessions were held in the afternoon (2pm to 4pm). Before each training session, the participants rested in the room for 5 minutes to have their blood pressure measured, followed by a general warm-up for the upper and lower limbs, consisting of general static stretches. At the end of each training session, the participants rested again for a new blood pressure measurement, with the aim of stabilising vital standards and being released. The RT programme was guided and supervised by a physiotherapist and two physical education professionals.

Table 1. Resistance training programme based on the Combined Series - *Bi-Set* with alternating segments. **RM,** Maximum Repetitions.
Source: Extracted from Prestes et al., 2010.

COMBINED SERIES - ALTERNATING BI-SET PER SEGMENT					
EXERCISES	RM		RM		RM
SEATED LEG PRESS	8-12		8-12		8-12
BICEP THREAD	8-12	Interval	8-12	Interval	8-12
EXTENSION CHAIR	8-12		8-12		8-12
SITTING SUPINE	8-12	Interval	8-12	Interval	8-12
FLEXURING TABLE	8-12		8-12		8-12
REVERSE FRONT PULLEY	8-12	Interval	8-12	Interval	8-12
SEATED LEG CURL	8-12		8-12		8-12
PULLY TRICEPS	8-12	Interval	8-12	Interval	8-12

CHAPTER 6

Training Protocol

At the end of the eight weeks of training described above, the participants were instructed to return to their daily lifestyles for the following eight weeks, but without any training intervention or physical activity, characterising the detraining phase. To control for the detraining phase, the participants were contacted weekly to ensure that the requirements for a sedentary lifestyle had been met.

CHAPTER 7

PROCEDURES AND DATA COLLECTION

7.1 Anthropometry and body composition

Although inflammatory markers can be influenced by adipose tissue (Sobieska et al., 2013, Tey et al., 2013), there was a concern to control this variable through anthropometric measurements and body composition. All the participants underwent the procedures in two stages Pre and Post eight weeks. Firstly, anthropometric measurements of body mass and height were taken to calculate the Body Mass Index (BMI) using a Welmy®-W300 digital scale with a maximum capacity of 300 kg and an anthropometric ruler with a scale between 1.00 and 2.00 m, as well as waist and hip perimetry to calculate the Waist to Hip Ratio (WHR) using a tape measure (Waist Fit ®). Body composition was then measured. Before the measurements, all the participants were instructed not to eat for 2-3 hours before the test, not to drink alcohol and not to exercise 24 hours before the test, to control their liquid intake and to urinate 30 minutes before the assessment. The participants were then asked to lie down on the stretcher to attach the electrodes to the predetermined points and sanitised with 70% alcohol. The emitter electrodes were positioned on the following sites: the dorsal surface of the right hand near the metacarpophalangeal joint, the distal region of the transverse arch of the upper surface of the right foot and the detector electrodes were positioned on the posterior prominence of the distal radius-ulnar joint of the right wrist and the other between the medial and lateral malleolus of the right ankle (Segal et al., 1998). This procedure was carried out using tetrapolar electrical bioimpedance (Maltron BF-906 Body Fat Analyser ®), whose technique is based on the fact that tissues with a high water and electrolyte content have a high electrical conduction capacity, while tissues with low water concentrations have a high resistance to the passage of current, which is a good predictor of body parameters (SIlva and Mura, 2007; Mcardle, Katch and Katch, 2003; Rodrigues, 2001). All these procedures were carried out at LAFIPEMA, UFMA and at two points in time, Pre and Post eight weeks, **Figure 3**.

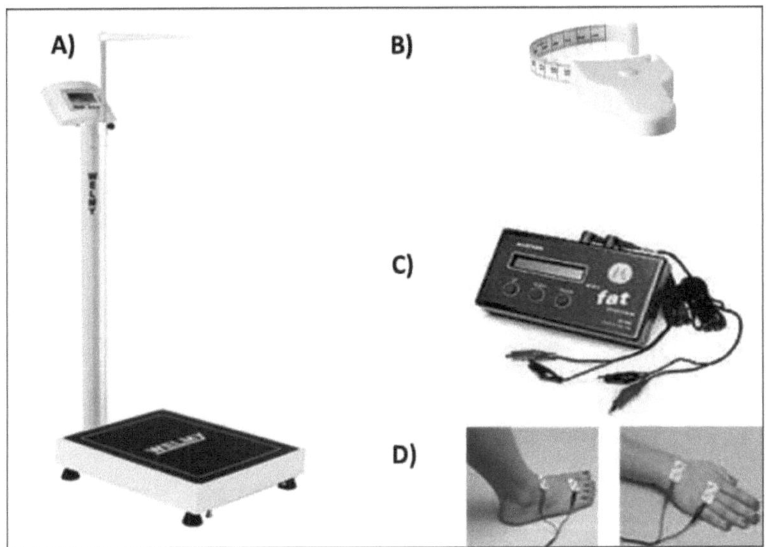

Figure 3 - A) Digital Scale (Welmy®-W300); B) Measuring Tape (Waist Fit®); C) Tetrapolar Electrical Bioimpedance (Maltron BF-906 Body Fat Analyser®); D) Positioning of the Electrodes.

6.1 Control of food consumption

In order to control and prove the regularity of eating habits for the group that received the intervention, all the participants in the TRAINED group answered a 24-hour Food Recall Questionnaire, Appendix 3, after each training session. This was applied by a previously trained nutritionist and consisted of a **checklist of the** number of foods, where the daily kilocalories (Kcal) of each participant were measured three times a week for a period of eight weeks.

6.2 Blood sample collection

Blood samples were collected by a trained phlebotomist and, in accordance with the biosafety standards recommended by NR32, samples were collected at two points in time, i.e. before and after 8 weeks. All the participants were told to turn up at LAFIPEMA, UFMA at 6am and to fast for a minimum of 8 hours and a maximum of 12 hours. The blood samples were collected under vacuum with a volume of approximately 14 ml, distributed in a 4 ml EDTA tube (**Vacuette**) and two dry tubes containing clot separating gel (**Vacuette) of** 5 ml each. The following measurements were carried out: a) the unit containing EDTA preservative was used to quantify the serum levels of the complete blood count (haemoglobin; leucocytes; basophils; eosinophils; lymphocytes; monocytes; neutrophils and platelets); b) the units containing the clot separating gel were distributed for the biochemical analyses of the lipid profile (TOTAL cholesterol, triglycerides, LDL and HDL-cholesterol), C-Reactive Protein. After collecting the blood sample, the tubes were labelled and transported in hermetically sealed thermal boxes to the Clinical Analysis Laboratory for biochemical parameters and the Laboratory of Immunology and Microbiology of Respiratory Infections - LAMIR-UniCEUMA.

6.3 Analyses of biochemical parameters

Biochemical analyses were carried out for the following parameters: a) For the inclusion criteria regarding alterations in the total number of cells that confirm infectious processes, a full blood count was carried out; b) For the control of fat mass through serum lipid levels, a full lipid count was carried out. c) For the control of serum levels of inflammatory markers, CRP analysis was carried out using the Immunoturbidimetry method, where the reference values, according to Pearson et al (2003) are: Low coronary risk: less than 1.0 mg/L; moderate: 1.0 to 3.0 mg/L and high: greater than 3.0 mg/L.

After blood collection, the biological material was transported to the Clinical Analysis Laboratory at UniCEUMA University for analysis. The measuring instruments for biochemical analyses were the SDH 20 and the LABMAX 240, **Figure 4**. The former is an automatic haemocytometer used to count blood cells using an automated photometry system with complementary microscopy. The LABMAX 240 analysed the complete lipidogram using the enzymatic colorimetric, homogeneous, selective surfactant and enzymatic methods for TOTAL cholesterol, HDL and LDL-cholesterol, triglycerides, respectively. PCR was carried out using the immunoturbidimetry method.

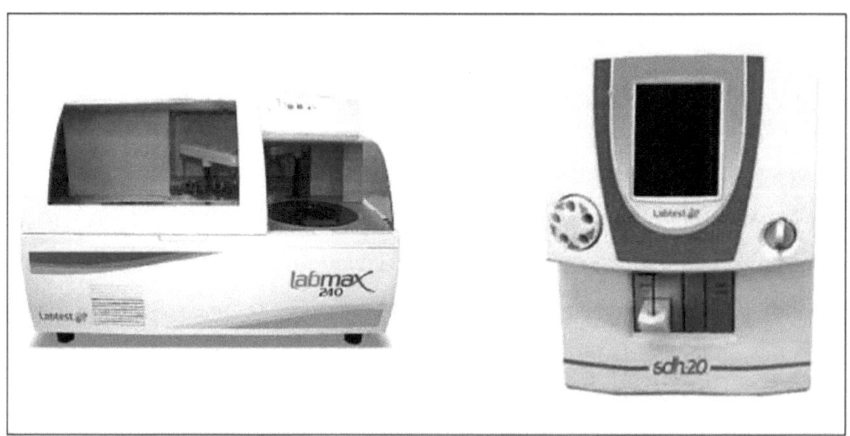

Figure 4 - Automatic haematology analysers (LABMAX 240 - SDH 20).

CHAPTER 8

Statistical analyses of the data

For statistical analysis, the data was presented (mean ± standard deviation). The Shapiro-Wilk normality test was then carried out ($p > 0.05$) for parametric tests. Group variables were presented as mean and standard deviation. For CRP, anthropometric variables, body composition and lipid profile at their respective times (Baseline, Post-Training and Post-Training), the ANOVA test (one way) was used followed by Tukey's post-test, as well as interaction and effect analyses between the samples. The correlation between CRP and anthropometric and biochemical variables was carried out using Pearson's correlation. The significance level adopted was $p < 0.05$. Statistical analysis was carried out using GraphPad Prism Software 6.0.

CHAPTER 9

RESULTS

When comparing the three moments (baseline, post-workout and detraining), we observed a statistically significant difference for the variables fat mass (p = 0.007), where it started at 27.1 ± 1.4 (baseline), decreased to 26.0 ± 1.3 (post-workout) and increased to 28.2 ± 1.8 (detraining).

On the other hand, lean mass showed (p = 0.0001), with initial values of 40.9 ± 1.2; increasing post-training to 42.0 ± 1.3 and a reduction in detraining of 40.0 ± 1.3. Next, the percentage of lean mass showed (p = 0.05) values of 60.1 ± 1.0; 61.73 ± 1.0 and 58.6 ± 1.2 (baseline, post-training and detraining). In terms of fat percentage, the three moments were 39.7 ± 1.0; a reduction to 38.2 ± 1.0 and an increase to 41.3 ± 1.3, respectively (p = 0.003). The same was true of total cholesterol (p = 0.04), with values of 192.90 ± 11.5, 152.4 ± 11.9 and 196.4 ± 14.6, respectively. The characterisation of the final sample at Baseline, Post-workout and Post-workout can be seen in **Table 2.**

Table 2. Sample characteristics and comparison between Baseline, Post-training and Dertraining.

Variables		(n = 9)	
Age		62 ± 2,3	
Height		1,54 ± 0,02	
	Basal	**Post-workout**	**Destreino**
Body mass (kg)	68,0 ± 2,3	68,0 ± 2,7	68,2 ± 2,8
Fat mass (kg)	27,1 ± 1,4	26,0 ± 1,3*	28,2 ± 1,8*t
Lean Mass (kg)	40,9 ± 1,2	42,0 ± 1,3*	40,0 ± 1,3|
Percentage of lean mass (%)	60,1 ± 1,0	61,7 ± 1,0*	58,6 ± 1,2*|
Fat Percentage (%)	39,7 ± 1,0	38,2 ± 1,0*	41,3 ± 1,3*t
BMI (kg/m)^2	28,4 ± 0,9	28,7 ± 1,0	28,6 ± 1,0
WHR (cm)	0,8 ± 0,0	0,8 ± 0,0	0,8 ± 0,0
Total cholesterol (mg/dL)	192,9 ± 11,5	152,4 ± 11,9*	196,4 ± 14,6f
HDL (mg/dL)	48,8 ± 3,3	50,5 ± 5,0	56,1 ± 5,3
LDL (mg/dL)	124,6 ± 11,4	112,7 ± 13,1	121,8 ± 24,1
Triglycerides (mg/dL)	107,8 ± 13,4	76,4 ± 12,5	102,8 ± 10,0

Data are presented as mean ± standard deviation. ANOVA test (p < 0.05).
* Statistically significant difference (p < 0.05) compared to Baseline.
f Statistically significant difference (p < 0.05) compared to post-workout.
BMI, Body Mass Index; WHR, Waist to Hip Ratio; HDL, High Density Lipoproteins; LDL, Low Density Lipoproteins.

In relation to the training schedule, the moments between the 1ª , 4ª and 8ª weeks of training are shown. It was possible to observe a progression of loads in their respective exercises with a significant difference between the weeks (p = 0.0001), **Table 3**.

Table 3. Training load evolution in the 1st, 4th and 8th weeks of the experimental group.

Exercises		Training Group (n = 9)		Effect Size	
	1ª week	4th week	8th week	(Δ)	p-value
Seated Leg Press (Kg)	20,7 ± 3,8	33,6 ± 1,1 *	45,4 ± 1,4 * f	6,3	0,0001
Biceps curl (Kg)	9,0 ± 1,8	13,8 ± 0,3 *	17,8 ± 0,4 * f	4,8	0,0001
Leg Extension (Kg)	9,9 ± 0,5	18,4 ± 0,6 *	25,9 ± 0,8 * f	28,0	0,0001
Bench press (Kg)	7,1 ± 0,3	13,8 ± 0,4 *	17,9 ± 0,7 * f	29,2	0,0001
Flex Table (Kg)	7,9 ± 0,4	15,5 ± 2,0 *	17,0 ± 0,5 *	22,1	0,0001
Inverse Front Pulley (Kg)	13,2 ± 0,5	21,9 ± 0,4 *	27,0 ± 0,5 * f	26,4	0,0001
Calf Leg Sitting (Kg)	20,0 ± 0,7	33,3 ± 0,9 *	43,5 ± 1,2 * f	30,9	0,0001
Triceps Pulley (Kg)	8,6 ± 0,6	16,4 ± 0,4 *	20,2 ± 0,4 * f	19,0	0,0001

Data are presented as mean ± standard deviation. *One-way* ANOVA test followed by Tukey's post-test.
* Statistically significant difference (p < 0.05) compared to 1ª week.
f Statistically significant difference (p < 0.05) compared to the 4th week.
Δ Measuring the size of the effect on the evolution of loads between the weeks analysed.

When comparing CRP between Baseline, Post-workout and Post-workout, there was a statistically significant difference (p =0.0001). The Tukey post-test showed a statistically significant decrease between baseline (2.0 ± 0.3 mg/L) and post-training (1.2 ± 0.3 mg/L), showing a (p = 0.008) and representing a 40% decrease in serum concentrations after the training phase. Between baseline (2.0 ± 0.3 mg/L) and off-training (1.5 ± 0.4 mg/L) there was a statistically significant difference (p = 0.02), representing a 25% reduction. When comparing serum concentrations between the post-training and detraining periods, the deleterious effects of detraining were not confirmed, but there was a 25% increase in the phase in which the eight weeks of training interruption occurred (detraining), where they are represented by the values from (1.2 ± 0.3 mg/L) to (1.5 ± 0.4 mg/L), (p = 0.4), **Graph 1**.

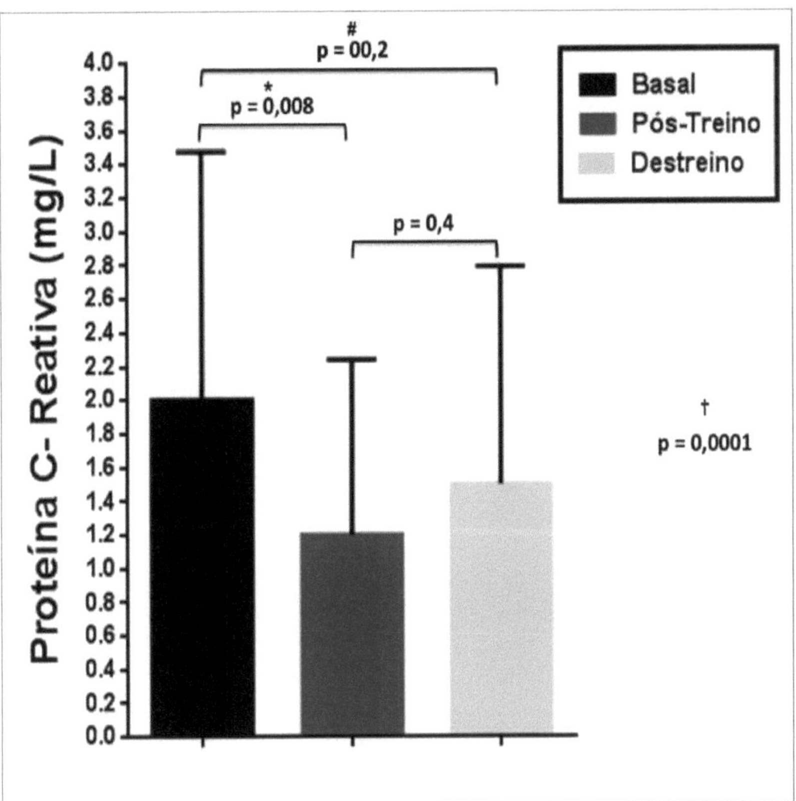

Graph 1. Comparison of serum C-Reactive Protein (CRP) concentrations at baseline, post-workout and during training in the experimental group (n=9).

* Statistically significant difference in Tukey's post-test of the post-workout moment compared to baseline.
# Statistically significant difference in the Tukey post-test of the Destreino moment compared to Baseline.
t Interaction and effect size between moments for the ANOVA test (one way).

When we correlated CRP with the other anthropometric and biochemical variables (Fat Mass, Lean Mass, BMI, Total Cholesterol and Triglycerides), we observed a moderate correlation between CRP and BMI ($r = 0.58$), followed by a weak correlation between CRP and the variables Fat Mass, Total Cholesterol ($r = 0.49$) and Triglycerides ($r = 0.37$). There was no correlation between CRP and lean mass ($r = 0.18$), **table 4 and figure 6**.

It is important to emphasise that the main anthropometric and biochemical variables were correlated with CRP.

Table 4. Correlation of moments (baseline, post-training and detraining) between the inflammatory marker C-Reactive Protein (CRP) and anthropometric variables and biochemical parameters.

Biochemical parameter	Fat mass (kg)	Lean Mass (kg)	BMI (kg/m)^2	Total cholesterol (mg/dL)	Triglycerides (mg/dL)
C-Reactive Protein (CRP) mg/L	r = 0.49 p = 0.009**	r = -0.18 p = 0.3533	r = 0.58 p = 0.001**	r = -0.49 p = 0.009**	r = 0.37 p = 0.053

**P≤0.01; *P≤0.05

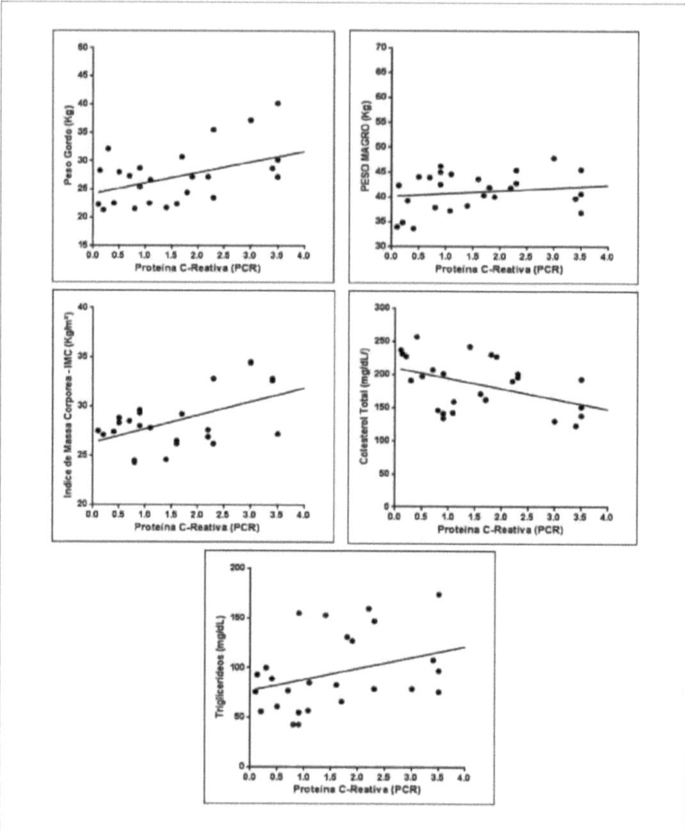

Figure 6. Graphical characteristics of the correlation analysis between C-Reactive Protein and anthropometric and biochemical variables.

CHAPTER 10

DISCUSSION

The aim of this work was to provide a scientific basis for the period in relation to the responses manifested in relation to training and detraining in the elderly. To this end, eight weeks of resistance training and detraining were analysed in relation to serum concentrations of C-Reactive Protein, body composition and biochemical parameters in elderly women. In this way, we can see that after 8 weeks of resistance training, the risk of cardiovascular disease decreased, represented by the reduction in serum CRP concentrations. In addition, we observed a reduction in fat mass and an increase in lean mass and training load, as well as a reduction in total cholesterol in elderly women. On the other hand, in the Training phase, we concluded that eight weeks did not significantly increase CRP, but it did negatively influence other parameters related to cardiovascular risk, such as anthropometric and biochemical values represented by an increase in fat mass and cholesterol, respectively.

Various systemic, tissue, cellular and molecular changes occur during ageing, with immunosenescence standing out, characterised by the progressive dysfunction of the immune system, with an imbalance in the concentrations of pro- and anti-inflammatory cytokines and other inflammatory markers such as C-Reactive Protein, which are associated with the development of cardiovascular diseases, increased co-morbidity and mortality in the elderly (Fagiolo et al. 1993; Pawelec & Larbi, 2008; Tonet & Nóbrega, 2008). Regular physical exercise protects against all causes of mortality, especially cardiovascular disease and type 2 diabetes mellitus (Petersen and Pedersen, 2005; Lee et al., 2014). Thus, some studies suggest that physical exercise is effective in reducing serum concentrations of pro-inflammatory cytokines (TNF-α, IL-1β, IL-8), promoting an **"anti-inflammatory" and protective** effect **in the elderly** (Córdova et al., 2011; Willis et al., 2012; Lee et al., 2014). Therefore, the systematic and progressive training of a RT programme is developed through appropriate and specific training goals. Among the various protocols used, the Combined Series - Bi-Set shows an efficient proposal for an individualised and well-structured RT programme that follows the recommendations for prescribing resistance training for the elderly, so within this proposal we chose to determine the intensity of the training by means of a zone of maximum repetitions between 8 and 12 RM, (AHA, 2007; ACSM, 2011; Tibana et al., 2012; Hyun-Sub Kim and Dae-Geun Kim, 2013). The results of this study suggest that chronic RT reduces biochemical parameters, represented by CRP and total cholesterol, as well as adipose tissue in elderly women.

A possible explanation for these events is that adipose tissue contributes to an increase in CRP concentrations, which results in an increase in serum concentrations (Akira, Taga and KIshimoto, 1993; Petersen and Pedersen 2005). Physical exercise induces a reduction in fat mass, where it mobilises lipids and stimulates lipolysis, which is regulated by lipase and activated by beta-oxidative stimulation, thus increasing the uptake and oxidation of fatty acids by skeletal muscle, serving as an energy substrate through the mechanism of the glucose-fatty acid cycle, directly reflecting a reduction in adipose tissue and, consequently a reduction in serum concentrations of acute inflammatory markers such as CRP and biochemical parameters such as total cholesterol, which is a beneficial event as it has a protective effect against cardiovascular diseases (Petersen and Pedersen, 2005; Silveira et al., 2011). The study by Willis et al. (2012) corroborates our findings, as they evaluated the effects of Aerobic Training, RT and Competitive Training over a period of eight months on body composition in overweight and obese adults and showed that Aerobic Training and Competitive Training tended to reduce fat mass. Another similar study was carried out by Ho et al. (2013), where they observed the effects of three training modalities (Aerobic Training, RT and Competitive Training) in participants aged between 40 and 66, followed up for 12 weeks and observed a reduction in fat mass and an increase in lean mass. Lee et al. (2014) monitored the effects of two types of training (Aerobic Training and Competitive Training) on body composition and biochemical parameters in elderly women over eight weeks and observed a reduction in fat mass and an increase in lean mass, especially in Aerobic Training. In terms of biochemical parameters, CT decreased serum concentrations of CRP and cholesterol compared to

AT. Based on the studies previously presented, we can speculate that the reduction in fat mass and increase in lean mass in our study were determining factors for the decrease in serum concentrations of CRP and Total Cholesterol in the elderly, since both are directly related.

In our study, during the Resistance Training phase, an increase in muscle strength was also observed, as evidenced by the progressive increase in training load and muscle volume over the eight weeks of training. According to Prestes et al. (2010), this episode is an adjustment by the body to training overload, with physiological (neural factors) and structural (muscle factors) changes occurring, resulting in an increase in muscle strength. The increase in muscle strength and volume can directly influence the decrease in serum concentrations of inflammatory markers (CRP), as these variables have a strong relationship with each other (Brito et al., 2011). Mavros et al. (2014) corroborate these findings, where they studied the effects of 12 months of RT on CRP in the elderly and associated their respective reductions with changes in body composition. The authors concluded that RT decreased serum CRP concentrations, as well as being associated with an increase in skeletal muscle mass ($p = 0.01$). In the study by Lera et al. (2014), they observed the importance of 16 weeks of RT on body composition, blood glucose and CRP in menopausal, sedentary and overweight elderly women and the results indicated that RT increased strength and muscle mass, as well as preventing an increase in glucose and CRP.

In the detraining phase, we observed that eight weeks of detraining was not enough to negatively increase biochemical parameters in CRP, but it did negatively influence other parameters related to cardiovascular risk, such as anthropometric and biochemical values represented by total cholesterol and fat mass. This study is of great importance for the clinical and practical aspects of exercise, as well as its interruption, because even when physical training is interrupted, the individual continues to benefit from the positive effects of exercise. For Fleck & Kraemer (2004), detraining is the result of a significant reduction or interruption in the volume, intensity or frequency of training, where the negative effects of detraining depend on the modality trained, the individual level of physical activity, age group and gender. In this way, the benefits caused by the metabolic and functional adaptations acquired through physical training play an important role in the organism of elderly individuals who maintain regular physical activity (Fleck & Kraemer, 2004 and Lee and coolaboradores, 2014). Otherwise, interrupting or reducing this regular activity could lead to a process of reversal of these benefits, resulting in significant increases in biochemical parameters and body composition, causing damage to health (Kraemer et al., 2002). Studies show that the increase in serum levels of metabolic parameters in the detraining phase is due to the triggering of an anabolic process as a reaction of the body to combat the catabolic process initiated by detraining, which is a harmful process for the individual, triggering a series of damages to the body (Kraemer et al., 2002; Nikseresht et al., 2014 and Tokmakidis & Volaklis, 2003).

With the reports cited, we did not observe significant changes in the detraining phase in relation to serum CRP levels in elderly women, leading us to reflect that eight weeks of training interruption was not enough to reduce these parameters, i.e. the elderly women were still under the effects of resistance training carried out during this period of time. This could be seen in the study by Rosety-Rodriguez et al. (2014) who analysed ten weeks of aerobic training followed by 4, 12 and 24 weeks of detraining in 20 obese premenopausal women (18-30 years old) and biochemical parameters (CRP). The training protocol was carried out on a treadmill (30-40 min), at a work intensity of 55-65% of maximum frequency, three times a week. The authors found that only from the 12th[a] week of detraining did these parameters begin to reverse, significantly increasing serum CRP levels, as well as the risk of cardiovascular disease. For the authors, CRP has a strong link with obesity represented by adipocyte cells, since the increase in inflammatory markers (TNF-α, **IL6 and CRP) would come from the production of** the adipocytes themselves and their degradation would lead to a reduction in inflammatory markers, including the risk marker for CVD represented by CRP. The authors conclude by reporting that when individuals interrupt their training programmes for a short period of time, they are still being influenced by the mobilisation and degradation of adipose tissue as an energy substrate, an effect known as lipolysis, so this mobilisation lasts for a few weeks, preventing a reduction in biochemical parameters such as CRP.

Another study that corroborates our findings was by Nikseresht et al. (2014), who analysed the effects of 12 weeks of training followed by 4 weeks of detraining in two types of training (non-linear resistance training and aerobic training) on CRP in middle-aged, obese men. The non-linear resistance training protocol consisted of 40-65 minutes of weight training with flexible periodisation. Aerobic training consisted of running on a treadmill at 80-90% of maximum heart rate. The study showed that there was no significant increase in serum CRP concentrations after 4 weeks of detraining. Nikseresht et al. (2014), as reported by Krogh-Madsen et al. (2002), explain that training induces insulin stimulation, which stimulates the expression of the IL-6 gene in subcutaneous adipose tissue in humans and that its stimulation reduces the number of adipocyte cells formed by adipose tissue, which is a beneficial mechanism for the body. During the detraining period, it will inhibit these factors, increasing body fat tissue and consequently inflammatory markers.

With regard to the increase in total cholesterol found after eight weeks of detraining in our research, a study published by Mann, Beedie and Jimenez (2015) addresses the negative events caused by interrupting training very well. On this occasion, the authors analysed the consequences of detraining, comparing an aerobic training (AT) protocol with resistance training (RT) on the lipid profile of diabetic individuals. A total of 30 individuals were studied, ranging in age from 45 to 50, all diagnosed with Type II Diabetes Mellitus and not receiving pharmacological treatment. They underwent 6 weeks of training, followed by 6 weeks of detraining. The participants were randomly divided into a TA group (65% of their maximum aerobic capacity) and a TR group (1 x 2 x 3 protocol at 65% of 1RM). The authors reported that both TA and TR indices improved during the 6 weeks of training, and during the detraining phase, these parameters worsened by increasing their values. The authors explain these positive and negative events with RT and detraining by reporting that the important role of RT is in relation to the metabolism of adipose tissue, especially fatty acids, because during exercise, lipolysis, stimulated by skeletal muscle in these tissues and regulated by hormone-sensitive lipase, activates the beta-oxidation of fatty acids derived mainly from triacylglycerides in adipose tissue and intracellular deposits in muscle tissue. This explains the efficiency and predilection of fatty acids as an energy substrate of active muscle through RT and the loss of continuity of training will occur the other way round.

Another study by García-Hermoso et al. (2014) showed the effects of 8 weeks of training followed by 8 weeks of detraining on HDL, LDL, total cholesterol and triglycerides in obese children and the overall results indicated that blood levels of HDL cholesterol and total cholesterol were increased in the detraining phase. As for the study by Parque and Lee (2015), who investigated the effects of 12 weeks of resistance training followed by 8 weeks of detraining on the lipid profile in elderly people with type 2 diabetes, they observed that the lipid profile was maintained after 12 weeks of resistance training, in the same way as in the 8 weeks of detraining.

Another important finding in our study during the eight weeks of detraining was the relationship between the negative changes found in body composition, where fat mass and fat percentage increased significantly. As mentioned above, physical exercise induces a reduction in fat mass, due to the mobilisation of lipids by stimulating lipolysis, and this event suffers negative changes during the detraining period (Petersen, Pedersen, 2005). In this way, the magnitude of the losses during the detraining period results from the intensity, volume and length of the training phase, which are determining factors for a readjustment in body composition (Hortobágyl et al., 1993). Thus, the study by Rosety-Rodriguez et al. (2014) corroborates our findings. The authors analysed the effects of ten weeks of aerobic training in 20 obese premenopausal women, followed by one, three and six months of detraining on body composition. The non-linear resistance training protocol was weight training, while the aerobic training consisted of treadmill running at 80-90% of maximum heart rate. The authors concluded that fat mass increased significantly in the detraining phase from the sixth month onwards.

Our study also found a decrease in muscle mass and lean mass percentage after eight weeks of detraining. The hypertrophy observed in muscle is associated with physical training and is regulated by hormones through mechanical muscle stimuli and occurs through local control (Bocca, 2015). Skeletal muscle disuse due to a decrease or interruption in the imposed overload leads to a decrease in the rate of protein synthesis and an increase in the rate of protein degradation, resulting in a decrease in muscle mass (Calura et al., 2008; Graves et al., 1988). Kraemer et al. (2002) reinforce this by reporting that in the process of detraining there can be a decrease in muscle mass due to a reversibility of the neuromuscular and hormonal adaptations that occurred during the period in which the individuals exercised. The study by Lovell et al. (2010) analysed the effects of sixteen weeks of strength training followed by four weeks of detraining on maximum strength and the rate of strength development in the elderly. The strength training protocol consisted of three sets of six to ten repetitions at 70-90% of one repetition maximum, three times a week. The authors concluded that 16 weeks of training increased muscle strength, isometric strength and muscle mass, however, after four weeks of detraining, all variables decreased significantly.

This study has some limitations that we should consider: a) We did not control the eating habits of the control group; b) In addition, there was a lack of specific tests to assess muscle strength. However, the results presented in the body composition with the increase in lean mass together with the increase in training load over the eight weeks, corroborated the conclusion that there was an increase in muscle strength in the population studied; c) There was no calculation of the power of the sample and the sample size of the study was considered **"small"**, however it was determined by convenience; d) There was a lack of specific tests (Cardiological and Glycaemic) to control the Exclusion Criteria, so a Directed Anamnesis was carried out to control this criterion; e) The representativeness of the sample, as it was a group of elderly women with a limited sample size and available to research an institutional care group. f) Another limitation of the study was that the elderly women had already gone through the menopause and it is known that the hormonal changes that occur in the postmenopausal period can be associated with cardiovascular risks, but it was observed that among some determining factors for this, such as a reduction in cholesterol and body composition related to fat weight, resistance training altered positively and in the detraining phase, the same parameters suffered negative changes with the interruption of training.

CHAPTER 11

CONCLUSION

Eight weeks of resistance training decreased serum concentrations of C-Reactive Protein in elderly women. In addition, there was a decrease in fat mass, an increase in lean mass and training load. In this sense, RT can be considered a non-pharmacological strategy for reducing inflammatory markers, as well as reducing risk factors for cardiovascular disease in elderly women. On the other hand, through the results found in the Training phase, it can be concluded that eight weeks did not significantly increase CRP, but did negatively influence other parameters related to cardiovascular risk, such as anthropometric and biochemical values represented by total cholesterol and fat mass. Finally, the continuity of physical training is essential for acquiring and maintaining good health, otherwise the beneficial adaptations achieved will regress to the initial values, and this depends very much on the type of exercise carried out, as well as the period of interruption in training.

Conflicts of interest

The authors declare no conflicts of interest.

REFERENCES

1. Abbas AK, Lichtman AH, Pillai S. Cellular and molecular immunology. Elsevier Editora Ltda. 7ª Edition Rio de Janeiro. 2012; 592.

2. ACSM - American College of Sports Medicine: Quantity and Quality of Exercise for Developing and Maintaining Cardiorespiratory, Musculoskeletal, and Neuromotor Fitness in Apparently Healthy Adults: Guidance for Prescribing Exercise, 2011.

3. AHA - American Heart Association: Cardiology and Council on Nutrition, Physical Activity, and Metabolism Update: A Scientific Statement From the American Heart Association Council on Clinical Resistance Exercise in Individuals With and Without Cardiovascular Disease. Circulation: Journal of

the American Heart Association. 2007.

4. Akira S, Taga T, and Kishimoto T. Interleukin-6 in biology and medicine. Adv Immunology. 1993; 54: 1-78.

5. Amaral PN, Pomatti DM, Fortes VLF. Physical activities in human ageing: a sensitive creative reading. RBCEH, Passo Fundo. 2007; 4; 1: 18-27.

6. Andersen LL, Andersen JL, Petter MS, Suetta C, Madsen JL, Christensen LR, Per A. Changes in the human muscle force-velocity relationship in response to resistance training and subsequent detraining. Journal of Applied Physiology, Washington, v. 99, n. 1, p. 87-94, 2005.

7. Barry BK, Carson, RG. The Consequences of Resistance Training for Movement Control in Older Adults. Journal of Gerontology: MEDICAL SCIENCES. 2004; 59; 7: 730-754.

8. Behrendt D, Ganz P. Endothelial function: From vascular biology to clinical applications. The American Journal of Cardiology. 2002; 3: 40-48.

9. Bocca Vieira de Rezende Pinto, Paulo Victor Sgobbi de Souza, and Acary Souza Bulle Oliveira. Normal muscle structure, growth, development, and regeneration. Current Reviews in Musculoskeletal Medicine. 2015 Jun; 8(2): 176-181.

10. Caldas CP. Ageing with dependency: responsibility and demands of the family. Cadernos de Saúde Pública, Rio de Janeiro. 2003; 19; 3: 773-781.

11. Cermak J, Key NS, Bach RR, Balla J, Jacob HS, Vercellotti GM. C- Reactive Protein Induces Human Peripheral Blood Monocytes to Synthesise Tissue Factor. Blood Journal. 1993; 82; 2: 51 3-520.

12. Coyle EF. Training and retention of training-induced adaptations. In: Blair SN, Painter P, Paite RR, Smith LK & Taylor CB. Stress testing and exercise prescription - American College of Sports Medicine. Rio de Janeiro: Revinter, 1994; 80-86.

13. Córdova C, Lopes-E-Silva F Jr, Pires AS, Souza VC, Brito CJ, Moraes CF, Sposito AC, Nóbrega OT. Long-Term Resistance Training Is Associated with Reduced Circulating Levels of IL-6, IFN-Gamma and TNF- Alpha in Elderly

Women. Neuroimmunomodulation. 2011; 18; 3: 165-70.

14. De Salles BF. Effects of resistance training on cytokines. International Journal of Sports Medicine. 2010; 31: 441-50.

15. Evangelista FDS, Brum PC. Effects of Physical Retraining on Athlete Performance: A review of cardiovascular and musculoskeletal changes. Revista Paulista de Educação Física, São Paulo, v. 13, n. 2, p. 239249, 1999.

16. Fagiolo U, Cossarizza A, Scala E, Fanales-Belasio E, Ortolani C, Cozzi E, Monti D, Franceschi C, Paganelli R. Increased cytokine production in mononuclear cells of healthy elberly people. Europe Journal Immunology. 1993; 23: 2375-78.

17. Fleck, SJ. & Kraemer, WJ. Designing resistance training programmes. 3rd edition. Champaign, IL: Human Kinetics Publishers, 2004.

18. García-Hermoso, M.D.a , M. Inés Carmona-López, M.D.a , José M. Saavedra, M.D.b ,and Yolanda Escalante, M.D. Physical exercise, detraining and lipid profile in obese children: a systematic review. Arch Argent Pediatr 2014;112(6):519-525

19. Gleeson M. Immune function in sport and exercise. Journal Applied Physiology. 2007;103: 693-9.

20. Ho SS, Dhaliwal SS, Hills AP, Pal S. Effects of chronic exercise training on inflammatory markers in Australian overweight and obese individuals in a randomised controlled trial. Inflammation. 2013; 36: 3.

21. Hyun-Sub Kim, Dae-Geun Kim. Effect of long-term resistance exercise on body composition, blood lipid factors, and vascular compliance in the hypertensive elderly men. Journal of Exercise Rehabilitation. 2013; 9; 2: 271-77.

22. Hsueh WA, Law R. The central role of fat and effect of peroxisome prolifereton-activated receptor-g on progression of insulin resistance and cardiovascular. 2003.

23. Kraemer WJ, Koziris LP, Ratamess NA, Hakkinen K, TRIPLETT-McBRIDE NT, Fry AC, Gordon SE, Volek JS, French DN, Rubin MR, Gomez AL,

Sharman MJ, Michael Lynch J, Izquierdo M, Newton RU, Fleck SJ. Detraining produces minimalchanges in physical performance and hormonal variables in recreationally strength-trained men.Journal of Strength and Conditioning Research. 2002; 16(3): 373-82.

24. Lazarim FL, Antunes-Neto JM, da Silva FO, Nunes LA, Bassini-Cameron A, Cameron LC, Alves AA, Brenzikofer R, de Macedo DV. The upper values of plasma creatine kinase of professional soccer players during the Brazilian National Championship. Journal Science Medicine Sport. 2009; 12: 85-90.

25. Lee JS, Kim CG, Seo TB, Kim HG, Yoon SJ. .Effects of 8-week combined training on body composition, isokinetic strength, and cardiovascular disease risk factors in older women. Aging Clinical and Experimental Research. 2014; 6.

26. Lera Orsatti F, Nahas EA, Maestá N, Nahas Neto J, Lera Orsatti C, Vannucchi Portari G, Burini RC. Effects of resistance training frequency on body composition and metabolics and inflammatory markers inoverweight postmenopausal women. The Jounal of Sports Medicine and Fitness. 2014; 3; 54: 317-25.

27. Lovell DI, Cuneo R, Gass GC. The effect of strength training and short-term detraining on maximum force and the rate of force development of older men. European Journal of Applied Physiology. 2010 Jun;109(3):429-35

28. Mann S, Beedie C, Jimenez A. Differential effects of aerobic exercise, resistance training and combined exercise modalities on cholesterol and the lipid profile: review, synthesis and recommendations. Sports Medicine. 2014 Feb;44(2):211-21.

29. Mavros Y, Kay S, Simpson KA, Baker MK, Wang Y, Zhao RR, Meiklejohn J, Climstein M, O'Sullivan AJ, de Vos N, Baune BT, Blair SN, Simar D, Rooney K, Singh NA, Fiatarone Singh MA. Reductions in C-reactive protein in older adults with type 2 diabetes are related to improvements in body composition following a randomised controlled trial of resistance training. Journal Cachexia Sarcopenia Muscle. 5: 111-120, 2014.

30. Melnyk JA; Rogers MA; Hurley BF. Effects of strength training and detraining on regional muscle in young and older men and women. European Journal of Applied Physiology, Berlin, v. 105, p. 929-938, 2009.

31. Mcardle WD, Katch FI, Katch VL. Exercise physiology energy, nutrition and human performance. Rio de Janeiro: Guanabara-Koogan. 2003: 1113.

32. Mosca L. C-reactive protein: to screen or not to screen? Engl Journal Medice. 2002; 347: 1615-7.

33. Mujika I, Padilla S. Detraining: loss of training-induced physiological and performance adaptations: Part I. Short-term insufficient training stimulus. Sports Medicine, Auckland, v. 30, n. 2, p. 79-87, 2001.

34. Mujika I, Padilla S, Pyne D, Busso T. Physiological changes associated with the pre-event taper in athletes. Sports Medicine, Auckland, v. 34, n. 13, p. 891-927, 2004.

35. Netto FLM. Biological and physiological aspects of human ageing and their implications for the health of the elderly. Pensar a Prática. 2004; 7: 75-84.

36. Nikseresht, M, Ahmadi, MRH and Hedayati, M. Detraining-induced alterations in adipokines and cardiometabolic risk factors after nonlinear periodised resistance and aerobic interval training in obese men. Applied Physiology, Nutrition, and Metabolism, 2016.

37. Nóbrega ACL, Freitas EV, OMAB, Leitão MB, Lazzoli JK, Nahas RM, Baptista CAS, Drummond FA, Rezende L, Pereira J, Pinto M, Radominski RB, Leite N, Thiele ES, Hernandez AJ, Araújo CGS, Teixeira JAC, Carvalho T, Borges SF, REH. Official position of the Brazilian society of sports medicine and the Brazilian society of geriatrics and gerontology: physical activity and health in the elderly. Brazilian Journal of Sports Medicine. 1999; 5; 6: 207.

38. Nonogaki K, Fuller GM, Fuentes NL, Moser AH, Staprans I, Grunfeld C. Interleukin-6 stimulates hepatic triglyceride secretion in rats. Endogrinology. 1995; 136: 2143-9.

39. Park SY, Lee IH. Effects on training and detraining on physical function,

control of diabetes and anthropometrics in type 2 diabetes; a randomised controlled trial. Physiotherapy Theory and Practice. 2015 Feb;31(2):83-8.

40. Papaléo NM. Gerontology: old age and ageing in a globalised vision, São Paulo: Atheneu, 1996.

41. Papaléo Netto M, Ponte J. R. Envelhecimento: desafio na transição do século. Atheneu, São Paulo. 2002: 3-12.

42. Pawelec G, LARBI A. Immunity and ageing in man: Annual Review, 2006/2007. Exp. Gerontology. 2008; 43: 34-38.

43. Pearson TA, Mensah GA, Alexander RW, Anderson JL, Cannon RO 3rd, Criqui M, Fadl YY, Fortmann SP, Hong Y, Myers GL, Rifai N, Smith SC Jr, Taubert K, Tracy RP, Vinicor F. Markers of inflammation and cardiovascular disease: application to clinical and public healthpractice: A statement for healthcare professionals from the Centers for Disease Control and Prevention and the American Heart Association. Circulation. 2005; 107: 499-511.

44. Persson GR[1] , Pettersson T, Ohlsson O, Renvert S. High-sensitivity serum C-reactive protein levels in subjects with or without myocardial infarction or periodontitis. Journal Clinical Periodontal. 2005; 32: 219-24.

45. Petersen AMW, Pedersen BK. The anti-inflammatory effect of exercise. Journal Applied Physiology. 2005; 98: 1154-62.

46. Petibois C, Déleris G. Effects of short and long-term detraining on the metabolic response to endurance exercise. International Journal of Sports Medicine, Stuttgart, v. 24, n. 5, p. 320-325. 2003.

47. Pedersen BK, Fischer CP. Beneficial health effects of exercise - the role of IL-6 as a myokine. Trends in Pharmacological Sciences. 2005; 28; 4: 15256.

48. Prestes J, Foschine D, Marchetti P, Charro M, Tibana R. Prescrição e Periodização do Treinamento de Força em Academias.Barueri, SP: Editora Manole Ltda. 2010.

49. Rodrigues MN. Comparison of body fat estimation by bioelectric impedance, skinfold thickness, and underwater weighing. Revista Brasileira de Medicina do Esporte , Niterói. 2001; 7; 4: 125-131.

50. Rosety-Rodriguez M, Camacho A, Rosety I, Fornieles G, Rosety MA, Diaz AJ, Bernardi M, Rosety M, Ordonez FJ. Low-grade systemic inflammation and leptin levels were improved by arm cranking exercise in adults with chronic spinal cord injury. Archives of Physical Medicine and Rehabilitation. 2014 Feb;95(2):297-30

51. Rossetti MB, Britto, RR and Norton, RC. Primary prevention of cardiovascular diseases in childhood and juvenile obesity: Anti-inflammatory effect of physical exercise. Brazilian Journal of Sports Medicine. 2009; 15(6): 472-75.

52. Santiago LAM, Neto LGL, Santana PVA, Mendes PC, Lima WKR, Navarro F. Resisted training reduces cardiovascular risk in elderly women. Brazilian journal of sports medicine 2015; 21 (4)

53. Santos Wellington Bruno, Mesquita ET, Vieira RMR, Olej B, Coutinho M, Avezum A. C-Reactive Protein and Cardiovascular Disease. The basis of scientific evidence. arquivos brasileiros de cardiologia. 2003; 80; 4: 452-6.

54. Silva SMCS, Mura JDP. Treatise on food, nutrition and diet therapy. São Paulo, Roca. 2007:112.

55. Silva FOC, MACEDO DV. Physical exercise, inflammatory process and adaptation: an overview. Revista Brasileira de Cineantropometria e Desempenho Humano. 2011; 13: 320-28.

56. Silva AO. Inflammatory, metabolic, anthropometric and body composition aspects in elderly women with and without insulin resistance. Master's thesis presented to the Catholic University of Brasilia, 2009.

57. Silveira L, Pinheiro C, Zoppi C, Hirabara S, Vitzel K, Bassit R. Regulation of glucose and fatty acid metabolism in the musculoskeletal system during physical exercise. Brazilian Archive of Endocrinology and Metabolism. 2011.

58. Smith LL. Tissue trauma: the underlying cause of overtraining syndrome? Journal Strength Cond. Res. 2004; 18: 185-193.

59. Sobieska M, Gajewska E, Kalmus G, Samborski W. Obesity, physical fitness,

and inflammatory markers in Polish children. Medical Science Monitore. 2013; 19: 493-500.

60. Ho SS, Dhaliwal SS, Hills AP, Pal S. Effects of Chronic Exercise Training on Inflammatory Markers in Australian Overweight and Obese Individuals in a Randomised Controlled Trial. Inflammation. 2013; 36; 3: 625-32.

61. Tey SL, Gray AR, Chisholm AW, Delahunty CM, Brown RC. The dose of hazelnuts influences acceptance and diet quality but not inflammatory markers and body composition in overweight and obese individuals. The Journal of Nutrition. 2013; 43: 1254-1262.

62. Tokmakidis, S. P.; Spassis, A. T. Volaklis, K. A. Training, Detraining and Retraining Effects after a Water-Based Exercise Programme in Patients with Coronary Artery Disease. **Cardiology**, Basel, v. 111, n. 4, p. 257-264, 2008.

63. Tibana RA, Pereira GB, Navalta JW, Bottaro M, Prestes J. Acute effects of resistance exercise on 24-h blood pressure in middle aged overweight and obese women. Internetional Journal Sports Medicine. 2012.

64. Tibana R, Balsamo S. Manipulation of the order of exercises in the prescription of resistance training. Revista Brasileira de Fisiologia do Exercício. 2011; 1; 10.

65. Tidball JG, Wehling-Henricks M. Macrophages promote muscle membrane repair and muscle fibre growth and regeneration during modified muscle loading in mice in vivo. Journal Physiology. 2007; 578: 327-36.

66. Tidball JG. Inflammatory processes in muscle injury and repair. American Journal of Physiology. Regulatory, Integrative and Comparative Physiology. 2005; 288: 345-53.

67. Toigo M, Boutellier U. New fundamental resistance exercise determinants of molecular and cellular muscle adaptations. Europe Journal Applied Physiology. 2006; 97: 643-63.

68. Tonet AC, Nóbrega OT. Immunosenescence: the relationship between leukocytes, cytokines and chronic diseases. Brazilian Journal of Geriatrics and Gerontology. Rio de Janeiro. 2008; 2; 11.

69. Xia D, Samols D. Transgenic mice expressing rabbit C- reactive protein are resistant to endotoxemia. Proc Natl Acad Sci USA. 1997; 6: 2575-80.

70. Willis L et al. Effects of aerobic and/or resistance training on body mass and fat mass in overweight or obese adults. Journal Applied Physiology. 2012; 113: 1831-1837.

71. Zaldivar F et al. Constitutive pro- and anti-inflammatory cytokine and growth factor response to exercise in leukocytes. Journal Applied Physiology. 2006; 100: 1124-33.

72. Zimmer. Socioeconomic status and health among older adults in Thailand: an examination using multiple indicators. Society Science Medine. 2001; 52: 1297-311.

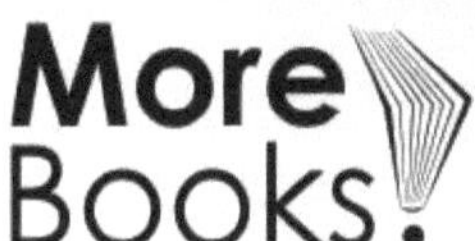

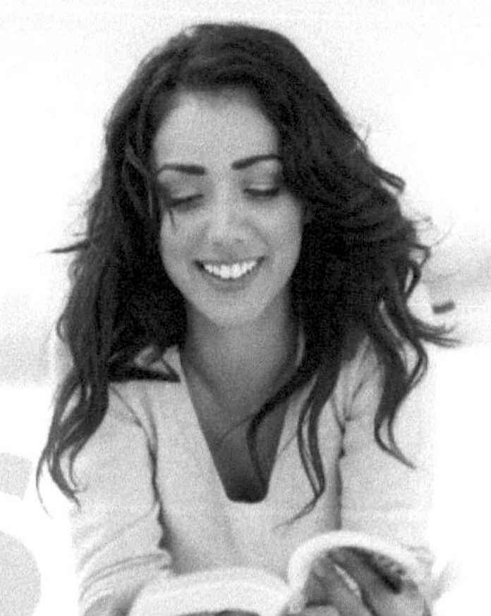

I want morebooks!

Buy your books fast and straightforward online - at one of world's fastest growing online book stores! Environmentally sound due to Print-on-Demand technologies.

Buy your books online at
www.morebooks.shop

Kaufen Sie Ihre Bücher schnell und unkompliziert online – auf einer der am schnellsten wachsenden Buchhandelsplattformen weltweit! Dank Print-On-Demand umwelt- und ressourcenschonend produziert.

Bücher schneller online kaufen
www.morebooks.shop

info@omniscriptum.com
www.omniscriptum.com

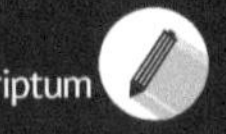

Printed by Books on Demand GmbH, Norderstedt / Germany